WILSON'S DISEASE MANAGEMENT DIET COOKBOOK

Nutritional Strategies For Wellness: A Comprehensive Cookbook–Balanced Eating For Health: Recipes & Tips For Wellness:

DR. SHAYLA LEWIS

Table of Contents

CHAPTER ONE 14
- What is Wilson's disease? 14
  - Causes and Risk Factors 14
  - Common Symptoms: 15
    - Diet is important for disease management. 15
  - How Can This Cookbook Help? 16
    - The Power of Nutrition in Managing Wilson's Disease 17
- Diet and Symptom Management 18
  - Importance of the Low-Carb Approach .18
  - Advantages of Antioxidant-Rich Foods .19
  - Anti-Inflammatory Diet to Manage Nerve Pain 20
  - Proper Nutrition Promotes Healing 20
  - Kitchen essentials for managing Wilson's disease 21
  - Stock Your Pantry with Nutrient-Rich Ingredients: 21
  - Essential Cooking Tools for Quick Meal Prep: 22

CHAPTER TWO 24

Tips for meal planning and batch cooking: 24
Understanding Food Labelling and Ingredients: 24
Food safety precautions: 25
How To Use This Cookbook: 26
Understanding Wilson's Disease: 26
Recipe Index: 27
Ingredient lists and substitutions: 27
Cooking directions: 27
Nutritional Information: 28
Variations and Customisations 28
Sample Meal Plans: 28
An overview of recipe categories: 29
Breakfast: 29
Lunches: 29
Dinners: 30
Snacks: 30
sweets: 30
Special Diets: 30
Tips for Tailoring Recipes to Individual Needs: 31
Dietary Preferences: 31

Texture and Flavour Preferences: 32

Meal Sizes: 32

Experimentation: 32

Sample meal plans for various dietary preferences: 33

Vegetarian Meal Plan: 33

Snack 33

Lunch: 33

Snacks include hummus and vegetable sticks. 33

Gluten-Free Meal Plans: 34

Snack: 34

Dinner 34

Low Sodium Meal Plan: 34

Breakfast: 34

Snack: 34

Lunch 34

Snack: 34

CHAPTER THREE 36

Common Concerns and FAQs 36

What is Wilson's Disease and how does it impact my diet? 36

What foods should I avoid to control my copper levels?..36

Are there any dietary guidelines that I should follow? 37

Can I still eat a variety of foods while controlling Wilson's disease? 37

How can I make sure I'm receiving adequate nutrients while following a restricted diet?...37

Interactions Between Medication and Diet 38

How do Wilson's Disease drugs interact with the diet?..38

Are there any food restrictions when using Wilson's Disease medications? 38

Should I take my meds with or without eating 39

Can dietary changes affect the dose of my medications? 39

What should I do if I encounter any side effects from my medicine or diet?..........40

Addressing Nutritional Deficits 40

Which nutrients are most typically inadequate in those who have Wilson's disease 40

How can I make sure I am receiving enough of these minerals in my diet?....41

Should I consider taking nutritional supplements...41

Are there any dietary components that can improve nutrient absorption? 41

How often should I have my nutritional levels checked?.......................................42

Managing Food Allergies and Sensitivities 42

What are the most frequent dietary allergies and sensitivities related to Wilson's Disease?...............................43

How can I know if I have a food allergy or sensitivity?...43

What should I do if I feel I have a food allergy or sensitivity?............................43

Are there any alternative items I can use in recipes to suit food allergies or sensitivities? 44

CHAPTER FOUR 46

Managing weight and blood sugar levels..46

Anti-inflammatory Meals for Symptom Management 46

Foods that reduce inflammation............47

Healthy Fats: 48

Fatty Fish: 48

Recipes for reducing inflammation and pain 49

Turmeric and Ginger Smoothie: 49

Quinoa Salad With Roasted Vegetables 49

Baked salmon with a herb crust: 50

Instructions: 50

Tips for Creating Anti-Inflammatory Meals 52

Prioritise entire Foods: 52

Embrace Variety: 52

Mind Your Portions: 53

Stay Hydrated: 53

CHAPTER FIVE 56

Meal Planning and Preparing for Busy Lives 56

The Importance of Meal Planning in Disease Management 56

Benefits of Meal Planning 57

Nutritional Balance: 57

Time Efficiency 57

Cost-effectiveness: 57

- Tips for Effective Meal Prep 57
  - Create a Weekly Menu: 58
  - Use Time-Saving Appliances: 58
  - Simple meals: 58
- Batch cooking for convenience....................59
  - Choose Batch-Friendly Recipes: 59
  - Label and Date Meals 59
  - Rotate Meal Selection: 59
  - Cool Meals Properly: 60
  - Use Freezer-safe Packaging: 60
  - Incorporate Variety: 61
  - Focus on Whole Foods: 61
  - Mindful Portioning 61
  - Consult a Dietitian: 61
- Delicious and Nutritious Breakfast Recipes 62
  - The Importance of Starting the Day Right: 62
  - Breakfast Recipes for Sustained Energy: 63
  - Quick and Easy Meal Ideas for Busy Mornings: 63
- CHAPTER SIX..66

Tips for Tailoring Breakfast Dishes to Your Taste: 66
Nourishing Lunch Ideas for the Go 67
   Packing Nutritious Lunches for Work or School 67
   Tips for Making Portable Meals. 68
   Adding Vegetables and Lean Protein to Lunches 69
   Healthy Options for Common Lunch Staples 70
   Delicious Dinner Ideas for Family Meals 70
   Importance of Family Dinners for Health and Wellness 71
   Dinner Recipes For Nourishment And Satisfaction 72
   One-Pot Meals for Easy Cleaning 73
CHAPTER SEVEN 74
   Tips to Make Dinner Time Stress-Free 74
   Getting Kids into Meal Preparation 75
   Delicious Snack Ideas for Anytime Cravings. 76
   The importance of healthy snacking: 76

Nutritious Snack Ideas for Any Taste Preference: 77

Portable Snacks for the Go: 78

Tips to Avoid Unhealthy Snack Traps: . 78

Adding Snacks to Meal Planning for Balanced Nutrition: 79

Delightful Treats for Special Occasions 80

The importance of balance in healthy eating: 80

Occasional threats that will not derail progress: 81

Healthy Dessert Recipes for Celebrations: 81

Tips For Mindful Eating On Special Occasions: 82

Balancing Indulgence and Overall Dietary Goals: 83

CHAPTER EIGHT 84

Dining Out and Socialising With Confidence 84

Navigating Restaurant Menus With Wilson's Disease: 84

Prioritise Fresh, Whole Foods: 84

Customising Your Order: 85

Strategies for Making Healthier Choices While Dining Out: 85

Plan Ahead: 85

Communicating Your Dietary Needs with Servers and Chefs: 86

Be Clear and Specific: 86

Express gratitude 86

Tips for Socialising Without Compromising Your Health Goals 86

Practice Mindful Eating: 87

Developing a Supportive Social Network for Healthier Living 87

General Principles 88

Conclusion 104

THE END 105

© 2024 Dr. Shayla Lewis All rights reserved.

No part of this publication may be reproduced, distributed, or transmitted in any form or by any means, including photocopying, recording, or other electronic or mechanical methods, without the prior written permission of the publisher, except in the case of brief quotations embodied in critical reviews and certain other noncommercial uses permitted by copyright law.

DISCLAIMER

Write a brief complete Disclaimer for my diet cook book telling them that the author is not in any association with any company, business or individual and also this book is written by the authors knowledge and understanding

The information provided in this diet cookbook is based on the author's personal knowledge and understanding. The author is not affiliated with, endorsed by, or associated with any company, business, or individual. The recipes and dietary advice contained within this book are intended for informational purposes only. Readers should consult with a healthcare professional or a registered dietitian before making any significant changes to their diet or lifestyle. The author assumes no responsibility for any adverse effects that may result from the use or misuse of the information contained in this book.

CHAPTER ONE
What is Wilson's disease?

Wilson's Disease is an autosomal recessive disorder caused by mutations in the ATP7B gene, which encodes a protein that transports copper from the liver to bile for elimination. This mechanism is hindered in people with Wilson's Disease, causing copper to accumulate in the liver, brain, and other organs. Over time, extra copper can cause significant harm to these organs, resulting in a variety of symptoms and consequences.

Causes and Risk Factors

Wilson's disease is primarily caused by genetic mutations acquired from both parents. However, not everyone with these mutations develops the disease, which is also determined by environmental circumstances and other genetic modifiers. Wilson's Disease, while uncommon, can affect people of any ethnicity or geographical region. Genetic testing can assist in identifying those who are at risk of acquiring the disorder, especially those who have a family history of it.

Common Symptoms:

Wilson's Disease can cause a variety of symptoms, which vary based on the amount of copper accumulation and the organs involved. Common symptoms include exhaustion, jaundice, abdominal pain, neurological symptoms such as tremors and dystonia, psychological symptoms like sadness and anxiety, and liver issues including cirrhosis and hepatitis.

Diet is important for disease management.

Diet is important in managing Wilson's Disease because it regulates the intake of copper and other substances that can exacerbate the condition. Foods high in copper, such as shellfish, nuts, chocolate, and organ meats, should be limited or avoided; foods that bind to copper, such as whole grains, legumes, and dairy products, can help reduce copper absorption. Individuals with Wilson's Disease should also maintain a well-balanced diet that promotes general health and liver function.

How Can This Cookbook Help?

This cookbook is intended to give delicious and nutritious dishes developed exclusively for those who have Wilson's disease. This cookbook attempts to make meal planning easier for persons managing the illness by focusing on low-copper foods that promote liver health. Each recipe is carefully designed to be both enjoyable and healthy for people with Wilson's disease, allowing them to enjoy flavorful meals while sticking to dietary guidelines.

To summarise, understanding Wilson's disease is critical for optimal management, and this chapter provides a complete overview of the disorder. Individuals with Wilson's disease and their carers can enhance their quality of life by learning about its causes and symptoms, as well as the relevance of nutrition in management. This cookbook is an invaluable resource that supplements medical treatment by providing realistic nutritional choices for people living with Wilson's disease.

The Power of Nutrition in Managing Wilson's Disease

Nutrition is essential in the treatment of Wilson's disease, a hereditary illness that causes copper buildup in the body. Individuals can greatly improve their health results by recognizing the complex interaction between diet and this illness. Patients can control their copper levels, alleviate symptoms, and improve their general health by making judicious dietary choices.

Wilson's illness necessitates a diet that limits copper intake while ensuring important nutrients are consumed. A well-balanced diet rich in vitamins and minerals is critical, with an emphasis on foods low in copper but high in nutrients required for metabolic function. This strategy not only helps to decrease copper absorption but also improves the body's ability to manage the situation properly.

Diet and Symptom Management

Diet is essential in managing the wide range of symptoms associated with Wilson's disease. Diet has an impact on more than just copper levels, ranging from liver dysfunction to neurological issues. Certain foods might worsen symptoms while others can improve them, emphasizing the need for dietary intervention in symptom management.

A diet customized to specific symptoms can help people feel better, improve their quality of life, and achieve better overall health results. Understanding how different nutrients interact with the body allows patients to make informed dietary choices that reduce symptom severity and promote well-being.

Importance of the Low-Carb Approach

A low-carb approach is extremely important in the therapy of Wilson's disease, owing to its ability to regulate insulin levels and reduce copper accumulation. Carbohydrates can boost insulin secretion, which promotes copper uptake in the liver and exacerbates the condition's symptoms.

A low-carb diet can help stabilize insulin levels, lowering copper absorption and alleviating symptoms of Wilson's disease. Individuals can improve their health and well-being by prioritizing foods high in key nutrients and low in carbs.

Advantages of Antioxidant-Rich Foods

Antioxidant-rich foods are extremely beneficial in the treatment of Wilson's disease, particularly in countering oxidative stress and lowering inflammation. Copper buildup in the body can cause greater oxidative damage, hastening the evolution of symptoms and consequences associated with the illness.

A diet high in antioxidants can help neutralize free radicals, protect cells from harm, and improve general health and vitality. Individuals can help control Wilson's disease by integrating antioxidant-rich foods into their diet, such as fruits, vegetables, nuts, and seeds.

Anti-Inflammatory Diet to Manage Nerve Pain

An anti-inflammatory diet has the potential to alleviate nerve discomfort caused by Wilson's disease while also increasing overall quality of life. Chronic inflammation is a typical symptom of the illness, which contributes to nerve damage and worsens pain and suffering.

Adopting an anti-inflammatory diet, which includes foods high in omega-3 fatty acids, antioxidants, and anti-inflammatory chemicals, can help relieve nerve pain and inflammation throughout the body. Individuals can effectively manage nerve pain and improve their general well-being by reducing inflammatory triggers and focusing on foods that promote healing and tissue repair.

Proper Nutrition Promotes Healing

Proper nutrition is critical for promoting healing and recovery in people with Wilson's disease, aiding tissue repair, and restoring normal function. The body requires a variety of nutrients to repair damaged tissues, regenerate cells, and promote general healing, highlighting the significance of a nutrient-dense diet in the treatment of the condition.

Individuals who prioritize foods high in key vitamins, minerals, and macronutrients can give their bodies the building blocks needed for healing and recovery. Proper nutrition is critical for patients with Wilson's disease because it supports liver function and promotes neurological health.

Kitchen essentials for managing Wilson's disease

Stock Your Pantry with Nutrient-Rich Ingredients:

A well-stocked pantry provides the foundation for wholesome meals. Choose whole grains like quinoa, brown rice, and oats, which provide critical elements such as fiber, B vitamins, and minerals. Plant-based protein and fiber can be obtained from a range of legumes, including lentils, beans, and chickpeas. Canned or dried fruits with no added sugars are a handy way to include fruits in your diet. Nuts and seeds include healthy fats, protein, and minerals such as magnesium and zinc. Finally, prioritize non-perishable foods such as canned veggies, low-sodium broths, and shelf-stable dairy alternatives to ensure a wide selection.

Essential Cooking Tools for Quick Meal Prep: Having the correct tools in your kitchen might help you prepare meals faster. Invest in high-quality knives for precision chopping and slicing. A collection of mixing bowls in various sizes makes it easier to assemble and store meals. A blender or food processor is useful for making smoothies, soups, and sauces. Nonstick cookware eliminates the need for unnecessary oil during cooking. Furthermore, kitchen gadgets such as a vegetable spiralizer or a rice cooker can increase the flexibility and convenience of your cooking routine.

CHAPTER TWO

Tips for meal planning and batch cooking:

Meal planning is an important method for keeping a healthy diet while treating Wilson's illness. Set some time each week to plan your meals, taking into account nutritional demands and personal tastes.

Batch cooking helps you to prepare bigger amounts of food ahead of time, saving time and ensuring that you always have healthful options on hand. Invest in meal prep containers to portion out meals and snacks for quick grab-and-go options all week. Experiment with recipes that can be easily scaled up and frozen for later use, ensuring you always have a choice of nutritious meals at your disposal.

Understanding Food Labelling and Ingredients:

Reading food labels allows you to make more educated decisions about the items you consume. Pay attention to serving sizes, as they can affect nutritional intake. Look for items that include a few additives, preservatives, and artificial chemicals. Choose whole foods and ingredients that you can pronounce, and avoid overly processed ones wherever feasible. Be wary of hidden sources of sodium, sugar, and trans fats, as these might increase Wilson's disease symptoms. When in doubt, pick fresh, whole foods and prioritize organic products to reduce your exposure to pesticides and other toxins.

Food safety precautions:

Proper food handling is critical for avoiding foodborne illnesses and ensuring that your meals are safe to consume. Wash your hands thoroughly before and after handling food, especially when working with raw meats, poultry, and shellfish. Keep raw and cooked foods separate to avoid cross-contamination. Use separate cutting boards and cutlery for raw and cooked foods, and sanitize all surfaces regularly. Cook meals at the proper internal temperatures to kill hazardous germs and pathogens. To maintain freshness and prevent deterioration, store leftovers in airtight containers labeled with the date.

Incorporating these kitchen necessities into your culinary repertoire allows you to control your diet while treating Wilson's disease. You can create a healthy kitchen environment by prioritizing nutrient-rich ingredients, using essential cooking tools, practicing effective meal planning and batch cooking, understanding food labels and ingredients, and implementing food handling safety precautions.

How To Use This Cookbook:

Welcome to the "Wilson's Disease Management Diet Cookbook"! This guide is intended to help people manage Wilson's illness by providing delicious and healthy dishes that are adapted to their dietary needs. Here's how to get the most out of this resource.

Understanding Wilson's Disease: Before getting started on the recipes, spend some time learning about Wilson's disease and its nutritional consequences. Consult your healthcare practitioner or a nutritionist to determine your individual nutritional needs.

Recipe Index: Browse the recipe index to find a variety of foods sorted by dietary preferences and constraints. Whether you're looking for breakfast ideas, main courses, snacks, or desserts, there are plenty of options to fit your preferences.

Ingredient lists and substitutions: Each recipe includes a full list of ingredients. If you have any allergies or intolerances, check the contents carefully and substitute as needed. Our "Tips for Adapting Recipes to Individual Needs" section offers advice on making suitable substitutes.

Cooking directions: Follow the step-by-step directions provided with each recipe. We want these directions to be clear and simple to follow, even for inexperienced cooks.

Nutritional Information: We recognize the importance of nutrition in managing Wilson's illness. That's why we've provided nutritional information for each recipe, such as calories, macronutrients, and micronutrients, to help you make informed diet decisions.

Variations and Customisations: Feel free to be creative with the recipes! Our "Making the Most of Recipe Variations and Substitutions" section provides tips for tailoring dishes to your preferences or dietary needs.

Sample Meal Plans: With some guidance, sticking to a healthy eating plan becomes easy. Check out our sample meal plans for a variety of dietary needs, including vegetarian, gluten-free, and low-sodium alternatives. These programs outline a strategy for balancing your meals throughout the day.

Incorporating dishes into Your Routine: Finally, make these dishes part of your daily food plan. Whether you're cooking for yourself or your family, these recipes are meant to be consumed regularly as part of a well-balanced diet.

We hope this cookbook is a helpful resource on your road to managing Wilson's disease with food. Bon appétit!

An overview of recipe categories:

We painstakingly handpicked a selection of dishes in "Wilson's Disease Management Diet Cookbook" to cater to varied tastes and dietary requirements. Below is an overview of our recipe categories:

Breakfast: Get your day started right with wholesome and energizing breakfast options ranging from robust muesli to protein-packed smoothies.

Lunches: Whether you're packing a lunch to go or having a leisurely midday meal at home, our lunch dishes provide a range of flavors and textures to keep you happy.

Dinners: From comfortable casseroles to bright stir-fries, our supper recipes are both delicious and healthful, making mealtime an enjoyable experience.

Snacks: Keep hunger away between meals with our variety of healthy and filling snack recipes, ideal for any time of day.

sweets: Satisfy your sweet desire with our range of guilt-free sweets made with healthful ingredients and delicious flavors.

Special Diets: We recognize that dietary restrictions differ from individual to person. That's why we've included a variety of recipes to fit different dietary preferences, such as vegetarian, vegan, gluten-free, and low-sodium.

Whether you're cooking for yourself, or your family, or entertaining visitors, our wide recipe collection will provide lots of inspiration. Happy cooking!

Tips for Tailoring Recipes to Individual Needs:

While our recipes are intended to be both delicious and healthful, we recognize that everyone's dietary requirements and preferences are different. Here are some recommendations for modifying our recipes to your specific needs:

Allergies and Intolerances: If you are allergic or intolerant to particular foods, such as dairy, gluten, or nuts, carefully study the recipe components and make any necessary changes. For example, you can substitute dairy-free milk for cow's milk, gluten-free flour for wheat flour, or seed butter for peanut butter.

Dietary Preferences: Whether you eat vegetarian, vegan, paleo, or keto, our recipes are easily adaptable to your dietary needs. For example, you can replace animal proteins with plant-based alternatives, use coconut milk instead of cream, or substitute cauliflower rice for regular rice.

Texture and Flavour Preferences: Feel free to modify our recipes to suit your tastes. If you like a smoother texture, blend soups and sauces until smooth. If you want stronger flavors, you can add more herbs, spices, or citrus zest to a dish.

Meal Sizes: Adjust your meal sizes based on your hunger and nutritional requirements. If you want to cut your calorie intake, you can lower portion sizes or bulk up your meal with more vegetables and lean protein.

Experimentation: Do not be scared to be creative in the kitchen! Cooking is all about experimentation, so feel free to adapt our recipes to your preferences. Who knows. You could find a new favorite meal along the way.

By following these guidelines, you can make our recipes fit effortlessly into your lifestyle while still eating tasty and nutritious meals. Happy cooking!

Sample meal plans for various dietary preferences:

Meal planning can be difficult, especially if you have Wilson's disease and must follow strict dietary restrictions. To make meal planning easier, we've produced sample meal plans for various dietary needs. Whether you're a vegetarian, gluten-free, or limiting your sodium intake, these meal plans give a foundation for creating balanced and delicious meals throughout the day.

Vegetarian Meal Plan:

Breakfast: Spinach and feta omelet on whole grain toast.

Snack: Greek yogurt and mixed berries.

Lunch: Quinoa salad with roasted veggies and chickpeas.

Snacks include hummus and vegetable sticks. Dinner is lentil curry with brown rice and steamed broccoli.

Gluten-Free Meal Plans:

Breakfast: Chia seed pudding and sliced fruit.

Snack: Rice cakes with almond butter.

Lunch is grilled chicken salad with avocado and quinoa.

Snack: Gluten-free crackers and cheese.

Dinner: Baked fish, roasted sweet potatoes, and green beans.

Low Sodium Meal Plan:

Breakfast: Overnight muesli with low-sodium nuts and seeds.

Snack: Fresh fruit salad.

Lunch: turkey and avocado wrap with carrot sticks.

Snack: Rice cakes and hummus

Dinner: Grilled prawns, quinoa and steamed asparagus

These sample meal plans are simply a starting point. Feel free to mix and match recipes to suit your taste and nutritional requirements. Remember to contact your healthcare physician or nutritionist to ensure that these meal plans meet your specific dietary needs. Happy eating!

CHAPTER THREE
Common Concerns and FAQs

During managing Wilson's Disease, several issues and queries may develop, often centered on diet, medicine, and lifestyle changes. Here, we answer some common questions to provide clarification and assistance to people dealing with this disease.

What is Wilson's Disease and how does it impact my diet? Wilson's Disease is a rare hereditary illness characterized by the body's inability to adequately metabolize copper, which causes it to accumulate in numerous organs, mainly the liver and brain. Diet plays an important part in managing Wilson's Disease by decreasing copper intake and promoting overall liver health.

What foods should I avoid to control my copper levels? Copper-rich foods should be limited or avoided, including shellfish, almonds, chocolate, mushrooms, and organ meats.

Furthermore, certain beverages, such as tap water from copper pipes, can add to copper absorption.

Are there any dietary guidelines that I should follow? Yes, following a low-copper diet is necessary. This entails eating foods low in copper while ensuring enough consumption of other elements essential for general health.

To design a personalized meal plan for Wilson's Disease, consult with a qualified dietitian who is experienced with the condition.

Can I still eat a variety of foods while controlling Wilson's disease? Absolutely! While some foods may need to be avoided, there are still plenty of delicious and nutritious options accessible. Include a mix of fruits, vegetables, nutritious grains, lean meats, and dairy substitutes in your meals.

How can I make sure I'm receiving adequate nutrients while following a restricted diet? It is critical to monitor nutrient intake and consider supplementation if needed. Working with a healthcare physician or dietician can help ensure that you satisfy your nutritional requirements while managing Wilson's disease.

Interactions Between Medication and Diet

Medication is frequently used in conjunction with dietary changes to treat Wilson's Disease. Understanding how these medications interact with your food is critical for improving treatment success and reducing risks.

How do Wilson's Disease drugs interact with the diet? Chelators (e.g., penicillamine, trientine) and zinc are two medications that might influence nutritional absorption and metabolism. Zinc, for example, competes with copper for absorption in the intestines, lowering overall copper levels.

Are there any food restrictions when using Wilson's Disease medications? Yes, certain foods or minerals can interfere with drug absorption and effectiveness. For example, high-fiber diets might impair the absorption of certain drugs, but dairy items may inhibit the absorption of zinc supplements.

Should I take my meds with or without eating? This is dependent on the exact medicine. Some drugs can be taken with meals to lessen gastrointestinal adverse effects, while others should be taken on an empty stomach for maximum absorption. It is critical to follow the instructions given by your healthcare professional or chemist.

Can dietary changes affect the dose of my medications? Yes, dietary changes, particularly changes in copper intake, can affect the dosage of drugs required to treat Wilson's Disease.

 Regular monitoring of copper levels and prescription adjustments may be required based on dietary changes and overall health state.

What should I do if I encounter any side effects from my medicine or diet? If you notice any concerned symptoms or side effects, such as stomach discomfort, appetite changes, or vitamin shortages, contact your doctor right away. They can assess your symptoms and make any required adjustments to your treatment strategy.

Addressing Nutritional Deficits

Nutritional deficiencies in people with Wilson's Disease might emerge as a result of dietary restrictions, drug side effects, or reduced nutrient absorption. Addressing these inadequacies is critical to sustaining general health and well-being.

Which nutrients are most typically inadequate in those who have Wilson's disease? Zinc, selenium, vitamin B6, and vitamin E are some of the most typically affected nutrients. Zinc deficiency is especially common due to its role in copper metabolism and its use as a therapeutic agent in Wilson's disease treatment.

How can I make sure I am receiving enough of these minerals in my diet? Consuming zinc-rich foods including lean meats, seafood, nuts, seeds, and whole grains can help prevent zinc insufficiency. Additionally, maintaining a varied diet that includes fruits, vegetables, and healthy fats might help with overall nutritional consumption.

Should I consider taking nutritional supplements? Supplementation with certain nutrients may be required if deficits are discovered by blood testing or dietary consumption is insufficient. However, before starting any supplements, talk with a healthcare expert to determine the optimum dosage and watch for potential interactions.

Are there any dietary components that can improve nutrient absorption? Yes, several dietary components can improve nutrient absorption. For example, eating vitamin C-rich foods alongside plant-based iron sources can improve iron absorption. Including healthy fat sources can also help with fat-soluble vitamin absorption, such as vitamin E.

How often should I have my nutritional levels checked? Individuals with Wilson's Disease must regularly evaluate their nutritional levels, particularly zinc and copper. Your healthcare practitioner might propose a blood test schedule depending on your specific needs and treatment plan.

Managing Food Allergies and Sensitivities

Individuals with Wilson's Disease may face difficulties managing their diet due to food allergies and sensitivities. Understanding how to identify and address these challenges is critical for maintaining a healthy and pleasurable diet.

What are the most frequent dietary allergies and sensitivities related to Wilson's Disease? While food allergies and sensitivities are not directly related to Wilson's Disease, people with this condition may nonetheless have them. Individual sensitivities may need the avoidance or limitation of common allergens such as nuts, shellfish, dairy, and gluten.

How can I know if I have a food allergy or sensitivity? Food allergies or sensitivities can cause a wide range of symptoms, including digestive difficulties, skin rashes, respiratory symptoms, and systemic reactions like anaphylaxis. Keeping a food diary and consulting with a healthcare professional might help you discover potential triggers.

What should I do if I feel I have a food allergy or sensitivity? If you feel you have a food allergy or sensitivity, see an allergist or immunologist for an accurate evaluation and diagnosis. They can do allergy tests and offer advice on how to manage your disease, including dietary changes if necessary.

Are there any alternative items I can use in recipes to suit food allergies or sensitivities? Yes, there are numerous substitute ingredients available to meet a variety of dietary needs. For example, nut allergies can be controlled by replacing seeds or seed butter for nuts in recipes, whereas dairy allergies can be treated by using plant-based milk replacements.

How can I avoid allergens while eating out or socializing? When dining out or attending social gatherings, it is critical to disclose your food allergies or sensitivities properly to restaurant personnel or hosts. To ensure a safe dining experience, inquire about ingredient lists, preparation techniques, and any potential cross-contamination hazards.

CHAPTER FOUR

Managing weight and blood sugar levels

Maintaining a healthy weight and stable blood sugar levels are critical components of controlling Wilson's Disease and improving overall health. Here are some techniques for accomplishing these objectives through food and lifestyle changes.

Anti-inflammatory Meals for Symptom Management

Understanding inflammation and its role in Wilson's disease.

In Wilson's Disease, a hereditary illness that causes copper to accumulate in many organs of the body, inflammation is a major factor in worsening symptoms and complicating treatment. Understanding the processes of inflammation allows people to adopt dietary choices that relieve pain and increase general health.

Inflammation is the body's natural reaction to an injury, illness, or irritation. In the setting of Wilson's Disease, inflammation is frequently caused by copper accumulation in tissues, which results in oxidative stress and damage. This inflammatory reaction can cause symptoms such as weariness, joint discomfort, liver malfunction, and neurological problems.

Foods that reduce inflammation

Adopting an anti-inflammatory diet high in nutrients that help reduce inflammation and promote general health is an important part of controlling Wilson's Disease. Adding the following foods to your meals can help alleviate symptoms and improve wellness:

Colourful fruits and vegetables are high in antioxidants, vitamins, and minerals, which help to reduce inflammation. Berries, leafy greens, tomatoes, and bell peppers are very effective in this aspect.

Whole Grains: Whole grains like quinoa, brown rice, and oats contain fiber and phytonutrients that have anti-inflammatory qualities. They also help manage blood sugar levels, which can assist in reducing inflammation.

Healthy Fats: Avocados, nuts, seeds, and olive oil are high in omega-3 fatty acids and other anti-inflammatory chemicals. These fats can assist in controlling the body's inflammatory response and promote cardiovascular health.

Fatty Fish: Fatty fish, such as salmon, mackerel, and sardines, are high in omega-3 fatty acids, which have anti-inflammatory qualities. Including fish in your diet a few times each week can help reduce inflammation and promote joint health.

Herbs and spices with strong anti-inflammatory qualities include turmeric, ginger, garlic, and cinnamon. Including these flavor-packed foods in your meals can boost their nutritional value while decreasing inflammation.

Recipes for reducing inflammation and pain

Cooking anti-inflammatory foods does not have to be complicated. Here are some easy yet delicious meals that can help reduce inflammation and manage symptoms of Wilson's Disease:

Turmeric and Ginger Smoothie:

Ingredients include frozen mango chunks, banana, plain yogurt, almond milk, turmeric, ginger, and honey.

For a refreshing and anti-inflammatory breakfast or snack, combine all ingredients and blend until smooth.

Quinoa Salad With Roasted Vegetables

Ingredients include cooked quinoa, roasted bell peppers, cherry tomatoes, cucumber, feta cheese, and lemon vinaigrette.

Combine all ingredients and drizzle with lemon vinaigrette for a healthful and anti-inflammatory lunch.

Baked salmon with a herb crust:

Ingredients include salmon fillets, breadcrumbs, fresh herbs (e.g. parsley and dill), lemon zest, and olive oil.

Instructions: Mix breadcrumbs, herbs, and lemon zest. Press onto salmon fillets, brush with olive oil, and bake until thoroughly cooked. Serve with roasted veggies for a filling, anti-inflammatory dinner alternative.

Adding Omega-3 Fatty Acids for Joint Health

Omega-3 fatty acids are vital nutrients that help reduce inflammation and promote joint health. Individuals with Wilson's Disease can benefit from including omega-3-rich foods in their diet to help control symptoms like joint pain and stiffness.

Fatty fish, such as salmon, trout, and sardines, contain the highest concentrations of omega-3 fatty acids, particularly EPA (eicosapentaenoic acid) and DHA (docosahexaenoic acid). These fatty acids have been found to lower inflammation in the body, which may alleviate joint discomfort and improve mobility.

For those who do not eat fish regularly, plant-based sources of omega-3 fatty acids include flaxseeds, chia seeds, hemp seeds, walnuts, and algae-derived supplements. Plant-based sources mostly contain alpha-linolenic acid (ALA), which the body can convert to EPA and DHA, but they also give significant anti-inflammatory properties.

In addition to including omega-3-rich foods in your diet, consider supplementing with fish oil capsules or algae-based omega-3 supplements to guarantee appropriate consumption of these vital fatty acids. However, before starting any new supplements, you should contact with a healthcare physician or trained dietitian, especially if you have underlying health concerns or are taking medications.

Tips for Creating Anti-Inflammatory Meals

Creating anti-inflammatory meals for Wilson's Disease requires careful preparation and decisions. Here are some pointers to help you create meals that support symptom management and boost overall health:

Prioritise entire Foods: Incorporate entire, minimally processed foods into your meals, such as fruits, vegetables, whole grains, lean protein, and healthy fats.

These nutrient-dense foods include critical vitamins, minerals, and antioxidants that reduce inflammation and promote overall health.

Embrace Variety: Include a variety of foods in your diet to guarantee you get a wide range of minerals and phytochemicals with anti-inflammatory qualities. Experiment with various fruits, veggies, grains, and protein sources to make your meals interesting and nutritious.

Choose Nutrient-Preserving Cooking Methods: Steaming, baking, grilling, and sautéing are better than frying because they help keep foods' nutritional integrity while reducing the development of potentially hazardous chemicals. Furthermore, utilizing herbs, spices, and citrus juices as flavor enhancers can give your dishes depth without using too much salt or bad fats.

Mind Your Portions: While nutrient-dense meals can help with inflammation, portion control is essential for maintaining a balanced diet and avoiding overconsumption of calories. To avoid overeating, pay attention to portion sizes and your body's hunger and fullness cues.

Stay Hydrated: Proper hydration is crucial for good health and can aid in the body's natural detoxifying processes. Drink lots of water throughout the day and avoid sugary drinks and alcohol, which can lead to inflammation and worsen symptoms.

By incorporating these ideas into your meal planning and preparation, you may develop a healthy and anti-inflammatory diet that helps with symptom management and improves your overall quality of life with Wilson's Disease. Remember to listen to your body, prioritize self-care, and seek personalized advice and support from healthcare experts or qualified dietitians as you work towards optimal health.

CHAPTER FIVE

Meal Planning and Preparing for Busy Lives

Meal planning and preparation become critical in the management of Wilson's Disease, where strict adherence to a specialized diet is required. This chapter discusses the importance of organized meal planning, providing practical advice and tactics to help those with busy schedules.

The Importance of Meal Planning in Disease Management

Managing Wilson's Disease requires rigorous adherence to dietary rules to control copper consumption. Meal planning is a proactive method to ensure that all meals meet these objectives.

Individuals who plan their meals ahead of time can more effectively control their copper consumption, avoid trigger foods, and maintain optimal health.

Benefits of Meal Planning:

Controlled Copper Intake: Meal planning allows for exact monitoring of copper content, which aids individuals in adhering to recommended limits.

Nutritional Balance: Meal planning that carefully picks ingredients can offer a balanced diet rich in critical nutrients while avoiding excessive copper.

Time Efficiency: Planning saves time in the kitchen by decreasing last-minute decision-making and the stress involved with dinner preparation.

Cost-effectiveness: Strategic meal planning can help people make more economical decisions, avoiding food waste and unnecessary spending.

Tips for Effective Meal Prep

Efficient meal preparation is essential for maintaining consistency in Wilson's Disease management diet. Here are some practical methods for streamlining the process:

Set Aside Dedicated Time: Schedule a specified time each week for meal planning and preparation, and regard it as a non-negotiable appointment.

Create a Weekly Menu: Plan your meals for the full week, taking into account dietary restrictions and personal preferences.

Wash, cut, and portion items ahead of time to speed up cooking on hectic weekdays.

Use Time-Saving Appliances: To make meal preparation easier, invest in kitchen appliances such as slow cookers, instant pots, and food processors.

Simple meals: Choose meals that are simple to prepare and need little cooking time, especially on busy days.

Batch cooking for convenience.

Batch cooking is a godsend for people with hectic schedules because it allows them to prepare huge amounts of food ahead of time and portion it for numerous meals. Here's how batch cooking can work for you:

Choose Batch-Friendly Recipes: Choose recipes that can be readily scaled up without losing flavor or quality.

Invest in Storage Containers: Purchase a range of airtight containers appropriate for freezing and reheating food.

Label and Date Meals: To ensure freshness and reduce waste, label each container with the contents and date of preparation.

Rotate Meal Selection: Keep a variety of batch-cooked meals in the freezer to avoid boredom and promote a diverse diet.

Freezing and storing meals for future use

Freezing foods enhances their shelf life, making them a useful option for hectic days when cooking from scratch is not possible. Follow these instructions to ensure safe and efficient freezing:

Cool Meals Properly: **To minimize bacterial growth, cool prepared meals to room temperature before freezing.**

Portion Control: Before freezing, divide meals into individual or family-size portions for simple reheating.

Use Freezer-safe Packaging: **Choose freezer-safe bags or containers to reduce the danger of freezer burn and preserve food quality.**

Thaw frozen meals safely by placing them in the refrigerator overnight or using the microwave's defrost setting to guarantee even thawing and flavor preservation.

Creating Balanced Weekly Meal Plans

A well-balanced meal plan is vital for satisfying nutritional requirements while effectively controlling Wilson's disease. Consider the following concepts while creating your weekly meal plan:

Incorporate Variety: **To guarantee proper vitamin, mineral, and macronutrient consumption, eat a variety of foods from each dietary group.**

Focus on Whole Foods: **Eat more whole grains, lean proteins, fruits, and vegetables while limiting processed foods and sugary snacks.**

Mindful Portioning: **Pay attention to portion sizes to avoid overconsumption of copper-rich meals while satisfying energy needs.**

Consult a Dietitian: **To personalize meal plans to individual needs and preferences, consult with a qualified dietitian who has expertise in managing Wilson's Disease.**

Individuals can manage Wilson's Disease while living busy lives by adopting meal planning ideas, efficient preparation procedures, and batch cooking.

Delicious and Nutritious Breakfast Recipes

Breakfast is widely regarded as the most important meal of the day, and with good reason. It establishes the tone for your energy, emotions, and overall well-being throughout the day. In this chapter, we'll look at the importance of starting your day with a nutritious breakfast and try out a range of delectable and nutrient-dense recipes.

The Importance of Starting the Day Right: Your morning routine can have a huge impact on your productivity, concentration, and even your weight management attempts. A well-balanced meal delivers critical nutrients and energy to your body and brain, boosting your metabolism and keeping you focused and alert.

Incorporating healthful ingredients into your morning meal sets a favorable tone for your dietary choices throughout the day.

Breakfast Recipes for Sustained Energy: To sustain consistent energy levels throughout the morning, your breakfast should contain a combination of carbohydrates, protein, and healthy fats. Muesli with nuts and fruit, healthy grain bread with avocado and eggs, or smoothie bowls loaded with greens and protein-rich components can deliver prolonged energy without the crash that sugary breakfast options are known to cause.

Quick and Easy Meal Ideas for Busy Mornings: Mornings can be hectic, but that doesn't mean you should forego a nutritious meal. Overnight oats, yogurt parfaits with granola and fruit, and whole grain breakfast wraps are all quick and easy to prepare in advance or assemble in minutes, making them ideal for busy mornings with little time.

Incorporating Protein and Fibre for Fullness: Protein and fiber are necessary components of a delicious breakfast that will keep you full and satisfied until your next meal. Incorporating lean protein sources like eggs, Greek yogurt, or tofu, as well as fiber-rich foods like whole grains, fruits, and vegetables, will help you suppress cravings and avoid overeating later in the day.

CHAPTER SIX

Tips for Tailoring Breakfast Dishes to Your Taste:

One of the pleasures of cooking is the opportunity to adapt dishes to your specific tastes and dietary requirements. Whether you enjoy sweet or savory breakfasts, have dietary requirements, or simply want to mix things up, there are numerous options for preparing delicious and nutritious breakfasts. Experiment with different ingredients, flavors, and cooking methods to personalize breakfast recipes and make each morning meal a memorable experience.

Understanding the significance of starting the day well and including delectable and nutrient-dense breakfast foods into your routine will set you up for success and provide you with a nourishing start to each day. Whether you prefer meaty and savory options or light and refreshing fare, there is a breakfast recipe for every taste and lifestyle on the following pages.

Nourishing Lunch Ideas for the Go

In today's fast-paced world, finding time to adequately nourish oneself over lunchtime might be challenging. Whether you're rushing to work or school, it's critical to prioritize balanced, nutrient-dense meals that promote your health and keep you energized all day. In this chapter, we'll look at numerous solutions and recipes for busy people who require nutritious lunches on the go.

Packing Nutritious Lunches for Work or School

When packing lunches for work or school, it's critical to prioritize nutrient-dense foods that give sustained energy. Choosing whole foods high in vitamins, minerals, fiber, and healthy fats will help you feel full and alert until your next meal. Incorporate a variety of fruits, vegetables, healthful grains, lean meats, and plant-based sources of nutrition into your lunchbox.

In this section, we'll go over practical strategies for choosing and cooking nutrient-dense ingredients, as well as innovative ways to put together balanced lunches that you can carry with you wherever you go.

Balanced Lunch Recipes for Energy and Focus.

A well-balanced lunch is vital for staying energized and focused throughout the day. By incorporating carbohydrates, protein, and healthy fats into your meals, you can assist in stabilizing blood sugar levels and avoiding energy dumps.

In this chapter, we'll look at several lunch recipes that will nourish both your body and your mind. From robust salads bursting with colorful veggies and lean proteins to filling wraps and grain bowls, there's something for everyone seeking for a nutritious and delicious lunch on the go.

Tips for Making Portable Meals.

Creating portable meals that are easy to take and consume on the go necessitates some forethought and imagination. This section will provide practical advice for preparing meals that are easy to pack and enjoy on hectic days.

From selecting the correct containers and packing procedures to combining fresh ingredients that retain their quality throughout the day, these suggestions will help you streamline your lunch preparation process and guarantee that you always have a nutritious meal on hand when you need it.

Adding Vegetables and Lean Protein to Lunches

Vegetables and lean meats are vital components of a nutritious lunch, as they provide essential nutrients and promote overall health. In this section, we'll look at how to incorporate more veggies and lean proteins into your on-the-go meals, including colorful salads, vegetable-packed wraps, protein-rich grain bowls, and stir-fries.

By focusing on plant-based foods and lean protein sources, you can prepare lunches that are not only delicious but also beneficial to your long-term health and energy.

Healthy Options for Common Lunch Staples

Many traditional lunch items, such as sandwiches, chips, and pre-packaged snacks, may not necessarily be compatible with your health and well-being goals. Fortunately, there are lots of healthful choices that are equally convenient and satisfying.

This chapter will expose you to healthy alternatives to common lunch staples including handmade whole-grain wraps, veggie chips, and good snack bars. These recipes and ideas will inspire you to improve your lunchtime routine by focusing on nutritional foods that promote your overall health and wellness.

Delicious Dinner Ideas for Family Meals

In the context of Wilson's Disease management, delivering good family dinners is more than just satisfying hunger; it is a foundational component of overall health and fitness. This chapter discusses the importance of family dinners, provides delightful recipes that nourish and satisfy, offers convenient one-pot meal options for fast cleaning, includes strategies for keeping dinner time stress-free, and investigates the benefits of incorporating children in meal preparation.

Importance of Family Dinners for Health and Wellness

Family dinners are more than simply a chance to refuel after a long day; they are an important ritual that promotes emotional connection, communication, and general well-being. According to research, eating together as a family has several physical, mental, and emotional health benefits. Sharing meals has a significant impact on both individual and familial health, ranging from increased nutrition and healthier eating habits to less stress and stronger family ties. Prioritizing family dinners for people with Wilson's

Disease can create a supportive atmosphere for dietary adherence and symptom management while also providing a sense of belonging and security.

Dinner Recipes For Nourishment And Satisfaction

Making nutritious and fulfilling meals is critical for people with Wilson's Disease, as dietary choices have an important role in treating symptoms and preserving liver health. This area has a carefully curated assortment of dinner recipes intended to provide maximum nourishment and satisfaction for the entire family.

From hearty stews and nutritious pasta dishes to tasty grilled meats and vivid vegetable medleys, each recipe strikes a balance between nutritional sufficiency and gastronomic enjoyment. These dishes, which incorporate a variety of nutrient-rich products and tasty seasonings, not only meet the dietary demands of people with Wilson's Disease but also appeal to the different tastes and preferences of family members.

One-Pot Meals for Easy Cleaning

In the rush and bustle of daily life, the notion of making lavish dinners might be intimidating. That's where one-pot meals come in handy, providing a quick and easy alternative for busy families.

This chapter features a variety of tasty one-pot dinner dishes that need little prep and cleanup, making them excellent for busy weeknights or idle weekends.

From substantial soups and savory casseroles to warm rice dishes and adaptable stir-fries, these recipes simplify the cooking process without sacrificing flavor or nutritional content.

By simplifying mealtime logistics, one-pot meals allow people with Wilson's Disease to prioritize their health without compromising time or energy.

CHAPTER SEVEN
Tips to Make Dinner Time Stress-Free

While family dinners can bring joy and connection, they can also be stressful and chaotic, particularly for individuals dealing with chronic health concerns such as Wilson's Disease.

This section provides practical advice and strategies for making dinnertime more joyful and stress-free for the entire family. These tips, which range from meal planning and bulk cooking to creating a relaxing environment and incorporating family members in meal preparation, attempt to relieve the stress associated with dinnertime routines. Families may turn stressful mealtimes into times of shared delight and nourishment by implementing effective mealtime habits and cultivating a positive dining atmosphere.

Getting Kids into Meal Preparation

Engaging children in meal preparation not only teaches them vital life skills but also promotes good eating habits and gives them a feeling of ownership and pride in their nutritional choices. This chapter looks at inventive methods to get youngsters involved in the kitchen, from simple duties like washing vegetables and stirring ingredients to more hands-on activities like assembling sandwiches and decorating pizzas. By making meal preparation a joyful and informative experience, families may help their children develop a positive relationship with food while also encouraging teamwork and cooperation.

For people with Wilson's Disease, involving children in meal preparation can be an excellent way to teach them about the importance of dietary control and liver health, setting the groundwork for lifelong wellness behaviors.

Delicious Snack Ideas for Anytime Cravings.

Snacking is frequently regarded as a guilty pleasure, but when done correctly, it may be an important component of a well-balanced diet, particularly for people with Wilson's Disease.

In this chapter, we'll look at the importance of healthy snacking, a variety of nutritious snack ideas to suit every taste preference, portable options for those on the go, tips for avoiding unhealthy snack traps, and advice on seamlessly incorporating snacks into your meal planning to achieve balanced nutrition.

The importance of healthy snacking:

Snacking is more than just a temporary delight; it is critical for maintaining constant energy levels throughout the day, reducing overeating at main meals, and ensuring that your body receives a consistent supply of necessary nutrients. Strategic snacking can help people with Wilson's Disease manage symptoms and improve their overall health. By selecting nutrient-dense snacks, you can increase your intake of vitamins, minerals, and antioxidants, all of which are essential for countering the condition's oxidative stress. Furthermore, healthy snacking can assist in regulating blood sugar levels, lowering the danger of unexpected energy dumps or cravings for bad meals.

Nutritious Snack Ideas for Any Taste Preference:

The key to successful snacking is variety. By incorporating a variety of foods, you can satisfy your taste buds while also meeting your nutritional requirements. There are numerous possibilities, ranging from crisp veggies with hummus to creamy yogurt parfait with fresh fruit. Consider incorporating a variety of carbohydrates, proteins, and healthy fats into your snacks to keep you feeling full and satisfied. Experiment with various flavors and textures to find your favorites, whether sweet, savory, or a combination of the two.

Portable Snacks for the Go:

Busy schedules frequently leave little time for sit-down meals, so portable snacks are a smart option. Stock up on travel-friendly snacks like mixed nuts, dried fruit, whole grain crackers, and individually wrapped cheddar sticks. Preparing snack packs ahead of time can help you avoid the temptation of vending machine delights while you're hungry on the road.#

Furthermore, investing in a high-quality insulated lunch bag or cooler can extend the shelf life of perishable snacks, allowing you to eat fresh, nutritious foods wherever you go.

Tips to Avoid Unhealthy Snack Traps:

While snacking has many advantages, it's important to be aware of potential drawbacks. Processed snacks heavy in refined carbohydrates, bad fats, and sodium should be avoided since they can cause inflammation and exacerbate Wilson's disease symptoms. Instead, choose whole, minimally processed foods whenever possible. Reading labels carefully and selecting foods with simple, easily identifiable ingredients will help you make informed decisions. Additionally, portion control is essential for avoiding excessive calorie consumption, so be conscious of serving sizes and avoid mindless nibbling.

Adding Snacks to Meal Planning for Balanced Nutrition:

Strategic meal planning can help you streamline your snacking routine while also ensuring that you acquire the nutrition your body requires. Consider including snacks in your meal prep by scheduling aside time each week to chop veggies, divide out nuts and seeds, and make homemade dips and spreads. When you have healthy options on hand, you are less likely to reach for convenience meals when you are hungry. To maintain consistent energy levels and avoid overeating, space out your snacks equally throughout the day, taking into account the timing of your big meals.

Understanding the benefits of healthy snacking, exploring a variety of nutritious options, and using practical success methods will allow you to enjoy great snacks while managing Wilson's disease.

Delightful Treats for Special Occasions

In the culinary road to managing Wilson's illness, one fundamental reality pervades every meal plan: balance. The precise balance between nutritional demands and occasional indulgence is critical for preserving not only physical health but also emotional well-being. Chapter 9 goes into the art of enjoying exceptional occasions without jeopardizing your nutritional goals.

The importance of balance in healthy eating:

Achieving and maintaining dietary balance is critical, particularly when dealing with a condition like Wilson's disease. It is not just about eliminating particular foods, but also about promoting a comprehensive approach to nutrition. Balance guarantees that you get all the nutrition your body needs while also leaving room for occasional pleasures. By achieving this balance, you can maintain your health without feeling deprived or overwhelmed.

Occasional threats that will not derail progress:

Contrary to popular perception, eating goodies on occasion can help you stick to your dietary plan. The idea is to choose snacks that are appropriate for your nutritional needs and interests. In this part, we look at a selection of indulgent options that won't derail your progress. From luscious desserts to savory pleasures, these carefully picked delicacies are intended to fulfill your appetites while keeping you on track for your wellness goals.

Healthy Dessert Recipes for Celebrations:

Who says desserts cannot be both tasty and nutritious? In this chapter, we present a range of scrumptious dessert dishes that are specifically customized to the dietary needs of people with Wilson's disease. From guilt-free chocolate truffles to refreshing fruit sorbets, these indulgences are not only delicious but also nutritious. Whether you're celebrating a milestone or simply craving a sweet treat, these recipes will satisfy your taste buds without compromising your health.

Tips For Mindful Eating On Special Occasions:

Special occasions frequently provide a plethora of tempting culinary delicacies, making mindful dining difficult to achieve. However, with the correct tactics, you may approach these situations with grace and intention. In this section, we provide practical strategies for practicing mindfulness on important occasions. From recognizing hunger cues to savoring each bite, these skills allow you to completely enjoy the pleasure of indulgence without overindulging.

Balancing Indulgence and Overall Dietary Goals:

Maintaining a balance between pleasures and overall nutritional goals is critical for long-term success. This final section delves into techniques for including occasional treats in your diet plan while remaining faithful to your nutritional goals. You can achieve the ideal balance of enjoyment and wellness by practicing moderation, paying attention to portion sizes, and prioritizing nutrient-dense foods.

By embracing the principles of balance, moderation, and mindfulness, you can enjoy the pleasures of food without jeopardizing your health goals. So go ahead and savor those unique times, and revel in the delight of feeding both your body and soul.

CHAPTER EIGHT

Dining Out and Socialising With Confidence

Dining out and socializing are important aspects of life that provide an opportunity for enjoyment and connection. Individuals with Wilson's Disease, on the other hand, may face distinct difficulties when perusing restaurant menus and social gatherings. This chapter will provide you with practical ideas and tips for dining out and socializing while staying on track with your nutritional demands and health goals.

Navigating Restaurant Menus With Wilson's Disease:

Understanding Menu Terminology: Learn about common menu phrases and ingredients that may be problematic for Wilson's Disease, such as high-copper meals like shellfish, organ meats, and nuts.

Prioritise Fresh, Whole Foods: Choose dishes that include fresh fruits, vegetables, lean proteins, and whole grains, which are often low in copper and provide a balanced diet for Wilson's disease management.

Customising Your Order: Do not hesitate to request menu item changes to better meet your dietary needs. Many restaurants accommodate particular requests, such as substituting high-copper products or changing cooking methods.

Strategies for Making Healthier Choices While Dining Out:

Plan Ahead: Before dining out, browse restaurant menus online to find suitable selections and plan your meal accordingly.

Portion Control: Be mindful of portion proportions, as restaurant meals are typically bigger than advised. Consider sharing dishes or ordering appetizers as main courses to effectively control portion proportions.

Choose side dishes that are appropriate for your nutritional needs, such as steamed vegetables or salad, over high-copper options like fries or creamy sauces.

Communicating Your Dietary Needs with Servers and Chefs:

Be Clear and Specific: Communicate your dietary limitations and preferences to waiters, emphasizing the significance of avoiding copper-rich items.

Inquire about how dishes are created and whether adaptations can be made to meet your needs.

Express gratitude: Thank the restaurant personnel for accommodating your dietary restrictions, encouraging positive interactions, and ensuring a nice eating experience.

Tips for Socialising Without Compromising Your Health Goals

Focus on Activities: Instead of focusing entirely on food, shift the focus of social gatherings to include activities such as walking, playing games, or visiting non-food-related events.

Bring Your Dish: Offer to bring a dish to social occasions that meet your dietary needs, providing you have a safe and delicious option to eat.

Practice Mindful Eating: Be aware of your eating habits and choices during social gatherings, savoring each bite and focusing on nourishing your body while still enjoying the company of others.

Developing a Supportive Social Network for Healthier Living

Educate Friends and Family: Taking the time to educate your friends and family about Wilson's

Disease and your dietary requirements will develop understanding and support.

Seek Supportive Communities: Join online support groups or local organizations dedicated to Wilson's Disease management to build a vital network of people who can offer advice, encouragement, and share their experiences.

General Principles

Steer clear of foods high in copper, such as whole grains, nuts, chocolate, mushrooms, shellfish, and liver.

Favor meals low in copper: Pasta, grains, white bread, fruits, and most vegetables are all dairy products.

If there is a lot of copper in the local water source, use filtered water.

Use glass, ceramic, or stainless steel cookware when cooking. Steer clear of copper cookware.

Weekly Schedule

Breakfast: Go for fruits, dairy, and cereals low in copper.

Lunch should consist of simple carbohydrates, safe veggies, and lean proteins.

Dinner is like lunch, but more varied to keep things interesting.

Snacks: Fruits, dairy, and high-nutrient, low-copper foods.

Day 1 of Week 1:

Breakfast consists of banana slices and Greek yoghurt with honey.

Lunch would be a salad of grilled chicken, lettuce, cucumbers, and low-fat dressing.

Dinner is white rice, steamed broccoli, and baked salmon.

Snack: A few slices of apple with a tiny bit of peanut butter

Day 2:

Breakfast consists of water-based muesli with blueberries on top.

Lunch is a white bread sandwich with turkey cheese and carrot sticks.

Dinner consists of a side salad (no nuts or seeds) and spaghetti with marinara sauce.

Snack: String cheese with less fat

Day Three:

Breakfast consists of a milkshake with strawberries, protein powder, and a scoop.

Lunch would be a mixed-vegetable quinoa salad (avoid the ones heavy in copper).

The supper will be grilled pork chops along with green beans and mashed potatoes.

Snack: A tiny bit of cream cheese on top of rice cakes

Day Four:

Breakfast consists of a slice of white bread and scrambled eggs with spinach.

Lunch consists of a chicken wrap with tomatoes, lettuce, and a low-fat dressing.

The supper will be baked cod over brown rice and asparagus.

Snack: pineapple pieces mixed with cottage cheese

Day Five:

Breakfast consists of mixed berries on the side and whole wheat pancakes.

Lunch is cucumbers, tomatoes, and lettuce paired with tuna salad.

Dinner is a stir-fried beef dish with white rice and bell peppers.

Snack: Slices of orange

Day Six:

Breakfast consists of a smoothie bowl with mango, yogurt, and a tiny bit of granola.

Lunch would be white bread and lentil soup.

Steamed carrots and quinoa paired with roasted chicken for dinner.

Snack: A little bit of cream cheese on celery sticks

Day 7:

Cereal with milk and a banana for breakfast

Lunch consists of cherry tomatoes on the side and egg salad on white toast.

The supper is pasta with prawns and a side salad.

Snack: Grapes Day 8 of Week 2

Greek yoghurt with strawberries and honey drizzled over it for breakfast.

Lunch would be a low-fat Caesar salad with chicken.

Dinner is sweet potatoes and green beans with baked salmon.

Snack: Sliced apples

Day Nine:

Breakfast consists of muesli mixed with raisins and a tiny bit of brown sugar.

Lunch consists of a white bread sandwich with gammon and cheese and carrot sticks on the side.

Supper is a stew of beef, potatoes, and peas.

Snack: String cheese with less fat

Day ten:

Breakfast consists of a milk, banana, and protein powder smoothie with a scoop.

Lunch would be a wrap with turkey and avocado.

Dinner is steamed vegetables and grilled chicken served over quinoa.

Snack: A tiny bit of cream cheese on top of rice cakes

Day Eleven:

Breakfast consists of a slice of white bread and scrambled eggs with spinach.

Lunch is tofu stir-fried with vegetables.

Dinner is baked cod served with asparagus and brown rice on the side.

Snack: Slices of peach with cottage cheese

Day Twelve:

Blueberry and whole wheat pancakes for breakfast

Lunch would be mixed greens and tuna salad.

Steamed carrots and mashed potatoes with pork chops for dinner

Snack: Slices of orange

Day Thirteen:

Breakfast consists of a yogurt, pineapple, and granola-topped smoothie bowl.

Lunch is white bread and chicken noodle soup.

Dinner is a stir-fried beef dish with white rice and bell peppers.

Snack: A little bit of peanut butter on celery sticks

Day Fourteen:

Cereal with milk and a banana for breakfast

Lunch consists of cherry tomatoes on the side and egg salad on white toast.

The supper is pasta with prawns and a side salad.

Snack: Grapes Day 15 of Week 3

Greek yoghurt with honey and a variety of berries for breakfast

Lunch would be a wrap with chicken Caesar.

Dinner is sweet potatoes and green beans with baked salmon.

Snack: A few slices of apple with a tiny bit of peanut butter

Day 16:

Breakfast is muesli mixed with apple pieces and cinnamon.

Lunch consists of a white bread turkey sandwich and carrot sticks on the side.

Supper is a stew of beef, potatoes, and peas.

Snack: String cheese with less fat

Day 17:

Breakfast consists of a milkshake with strawberries, protein powder, and a scoop.

Lunch would be a wrap with cheese and ham.

Dinner is steamed vegetables and grilled chicken served over quinoa.

Snack: A tiny bit of cream cheese on top of rice cakes

Day 18:

Breakfast consists of a slice of white bread and scrambled eggs with spinach.

Lunch is tofu stir-fried with vegetables.

Dinner is baked cod served with asparagus and brown rice on the side.

Snack: pineapple pieces mixed with cottage cheese

Day 19:

Breakfast consists of mixed berries on the side and whole wheat pancakes.

Lunch would be mixed greens and tuna salad.

Steamed carrots and mashed potatoes with pork chops for dinner

Snack: Slices of orange

Day 20:

Breakfast consists of a smoothie bowl with mango, yogurt, and a tiny bit of granola.

Lunch is white bread and chicken noodle soup.

Dinner is a stir-fried beef dish with white rice and bell peppers.

Snack: A little bit of cream cheese on celery sticks

Day 21:

Cereal with milk and a banana for breakfast

Lunch consists of cherry tomatoes on the side and egg salad on white toast.

The supper is pasta with prawns and a side salad.

Snack: Grapes Day 22 of Week 4

Greek yoghurt with honey and a variety of berries for breakfast

Lunch would be a wrap with chicken Caesar.

Dinner is sweet potatoes and green beans with baked salmon.

Snack: Sliced apples

Day 23:

Breakfast is muesli mixed with apple pieces and cinnamon.

Lunch consists of a white bread turkey sandwich and carrot sticks on the side.

Supper is a stew of beef, potatoes, and peas.

Snack: String cheese with less fat

Day 24:

Breakfast consists of a milkshake with strawberries, protein powder, and a scoop.

Lunch would be a wrap with cheese and ham.

Dinner is steamed vegetables and grilled chicken served over quinoa.

Snack: A tiny bit of cream cheese on top of rice cakes

Day 25:

Breakfast consists of a slice of white bread and scrambled eggs with spinach.

Lunch is tofu stir-fried with vegetables.

Dinner is baked cod served with asparagus and brown rice on the side.

Snack: Slices of peach with cottage cheese

Day 26:

Blueberry and whole wheat pancakes for breakfast

Lunch would be mixed greens and tuna salad.

Steamed carrots and mashed potatoes with pork chops for dinner

Snack: Slices of orange

Day 27:

Breakfast consists of a yogurt, pineapple, and granola-topped smoothie bowl.

Lunch is white bread and chicken noodle soup.

Dinner is a stir-fried beef dish with white rice and bell peppers.

Snack: A little bit of peanut butter on celery sticks

Day 28:

Cereal with milk and a banana for breakfast

Lunch consists of cherry tomatoes on the side and egg salad on white toast.

The supper is pasta with prawns and a side salad.

Snack: Grapes Day 29 of Week 5

Greek yoghurt with honey and a variety of berries for breakfast

Lunch would be a wrap with chicken Caesar.

Dinner is sweet potatoes and green beans with baked salmon.

Snack: A few slices of apple with a tiny bit of peanut butter

Day 30:

Breakfast is muesli mixed with apple pieces and cinnamon.

Lunch consists of a white bread turkey sandwich and carrot sticks on the side.

Supper is a stew of beef, potatoes, and peas.

Snack: String cheese with less fat

Conclusion: Even if you are managing Wilson's Disease, dining out and socializing may be pleasurable and rewarding experiences. You may confidently negotiate these situations while prioritizing your health goals by using practical tactics, excellent communication, and developing a supporting social network. Stay informed, advocate for your needs, and enjoy the company of friends and loved ones as you embark on your wellness journey.

THE END

www.ingramcontent.com/pod-product-compliance
Lightning Source LLC
Chambersburg PA
CBHW052330220526
45472CB00001B/349